BEGINNERS GUIDE ON KELOIDS

A Simple Guide on Keloid Treatment and Management

Ana Todd

Chapter one

What are keloids?

Keloids are raised scar. They appear where the skin has healed after an injury. They have the potential to become much larger than the original injury that caused the scar. They are extremely rare, but are more common for people with dark complexion.

A keloid could the result by anything that can generate a scar. This includes being burnt, cut, or suffering from severe acne. Keloids can also develop as a result of a body piercing, tattoo, or surgery. Keloids might appear 3months or more after your skin had been wounded. Some will still continue growing for years.

History of Keloids

Regarding surgical procedures, Egyptian surgeons mentioned keloids circa 1700 BC in the Smith papyrus. In 1806 Baron Jean-Louis Alibert (1768-1837) defined the keloid as a distinct organism. He named them cancroide, but later changed it to chélode to prevent confusion with cancer. The word is derived from the Ancient Greek chele, which means "crab pincers," and the suffix -oid, which means "like."

The iconic American Civil War-era portrait "Whipped Peter" depicts an escaped former slave with extensive keloid scars from his former overseer's brutal beatings.

Intralesional corticosteroid injections were first used as a treatment to attenuate scarring in the mid-1960s. Since the 1970s, pressure therapy has been used to prevent and treat keloids.

In the early 1980s, topical silicone gel sheeting was introduced as a therapy.

Keloids Symptoms

Keloids can have the following characteristics.

- **They Appear and Grow Slowly:** The initial signs of a keloid might appear anywhere between three months and a year. It then takes weeks or months to grow. They may sometimes grow slowly for years.

- **It all starts with a raised pink, red, or purple scar:** Keloid scars are often raised scars with a flat surface. With time, the color darkens. It is usually darker than the person's complexion, with the border darker than the center.

- **Feel different from the surrounding skin:** Some keloids have a soft, doughy texture. Others are harder and rubbery.

- **Cause discomfort, itching, or tenderness:** Some keloids may be itchy, irritating, or unpleasant to the touch while forming. These symptoms normally go away once the keloid has stopped growing.

Keloids can grow in any part of the body. They are most frequently found on the neck, shoulders, chest, back, and ears.

They could be as tiny as an inch or as big as 12 inches or more.

Causes of keloids

When you injure your skin, your cells attempt to repair it by forming a scar. Scar tissue still continues to grow in some people even after the wound has been healed. The raised area on your skin is caused by the excess scar tissue. Doctors are still baffled as to why certain people skin scars in this manner.

A keloid can develop from a variety of skin injuries. This includes

- Cuts

- puncture wounds
- surgical scars
- severe acne
- chicken pox
- insect bites
- injection sites
- piercings
- tattoos

When some people scar, they are more likely to produce a keloid. You are more prone to develop a keloid if you are:

- Black, Latino, or Asian.
- You are below 30 years old.
- Pregnant.
- An adolescent going through puberty.

- You have a family background of keloids.

Darker skinned people are 15% to 20% more prone to develop keloids.

How are Keloids Diagnosed

A keloid can be identified by your doctor based on the raised scar on your skin. He or she may occasionally perform a skin biopsy to rule out other types of skin growths.

Can keloids be Avoided or Prevented?

People who are likely to have keloids may choose not to undergo a body piercing or tattoo. If you get your ears pierced, wear pressure earrings to prevent scarring on your earlobes.

Chapter Two

Treatment

The treatment's goal is to flatten, soften, or decrease the raised scar. Keloids might be difficult to get rid of. They sometimes reappear after treatment. Many doctors will combine treatment to achieve the best outcomes. The following treatments are available:

- **Corticosteroid injections.** The medicine in these shots aids in scar shrinking.
- **Cryotherapy**. Applying ice to the scar or cold therapy, can be used to soften and

shrink scars. It is more effective on small keloids.

- **Wearing silicone sheets or gel on the scar**. This can help in flattening of the keloid.

- **Laser Therapy**. This can aid flattening of the keloid. It might also fade the color.

- **Surgical Removal**. This entails cutting the keloid. The majority of keloids will return after this treatment.

- **Pressure Treatment.** Maintaining pressure on the area after keloid surgery reduces blood flow. This can help to keep a keloid from recurring.

Keloids Home Remedies

The best strategy for dealing with keloid-prone skin is generally seen to be prevention. The following home remedies may help in wound healing and preventing keloid development from a scar:

- **Aspirin:** Making a paste of crushed aspirin pills and applying it to the scar for one or two hours may help minimize scars that appear larger or darker due to inflammation.
- **Honey:** Due to its anti-inflammatory properties, honey is used in a variety of

skin treatments and wound dressings. It can aid in the reduction of scar size and appearance. Certain types of honey, such as Kelulut honey (a honey with strong antioxidant qualities), have been found to be more potent and probably more effective than others.

- **Garlic:** Garlic has been used as a home remedy for wound healing and infection prevention for centuries. Several studies have indicated that using garlic extract topically can help prevent and cure scarring. Allicin is the primary ingredient that is said to help lighten and reduce the size of scars while also improving healing.

- **Onion:** Extracts from onion, which is often sold as a topical ointment (Cepalin), has an anti-inflammatory properties that helps in prevent the formation of scar tissue. According to some experts, onion is the next best thing to silicone-based scar prevention solutions.

NOTE: Different treatments are effective for different persons. Consult your doctor to determine

which treatment choice is best for
you.

Chapter Three

Living with Keloids

Keloids are not dangerous to your health, although they can be upsetting. You might sometimes be embarrassed by how they look. This can be detrimental to your self-esteem. Most people seek therapy for keloids because they dislike their appearance. Fortunately, existing therapies can enhance the appearance of keloids even if they do not entirely remove the scars.

Ways to Boost Your Self-Esteem

If you have keloid-prone skin, the likelihood of one of these scars appearing on a visible part of your body is considerable high. Researchers discovered that 40% of persons with exposed keloid scars felt that their scars had a negative impact on their self-image in a study of 61 people.

Physical signs of a keloid include itching, movement limitations, and other discomforts. These scars can also cause psychosocial effect such as depression, anxiety, and other daily stresses.

A healthcare provider or therapist can assist you in managing your impression of scarring, particularly in highly visible areas. Knowing your keloid risk and how to reduce excessive scarring will help you cope.

Other Coping Strategies of Keloids

- Find a support group or a community of individuals who share your situation.
- Think about cognitive behavioral therapy (a type of talk therapy) to evaluate and improve dysfunctional beliefs and self-assumptions and aid in decision-making,

overcoming social anxiety, and enhancing self-worth.

- Consider counseling or meditation to help you cope with anxiety or concern about your appearance.

Quick Facts about Keloids:

- Keloids can be a concern owing to their appearance, especially if they appear on the face, neck, or hands.
- There is no perfect method for removing keloids.
- Prescription medications and in-office procedures may be able to enhance the appearance of keloids.

How Long Will The Keloid Take To Disappear?

"Keloids cannot be completely removed," says Dr. Harish Koutam, principal dermatologist at SkinKraft Laboratories. The time it takes to diminish it will depend on the size of the keloid and the treatment approach you choose."

For example, if you had a keloid bump surgically excision, it would be gone in one go. However, if other treatments are not used, it may return sooner or later. Laser therapy or steroid injections will require numerous sessions to completely remove the scar.

How Can You Prevent Keloid from Growing?

- If you are prone to keloid formation, avoid cosmetic surgical operations, tattooing, body piercing, and so on.
- In the event of an unavoidable injury, begin treating the injured region as soon as possible to expedite the healing process. Clean the wound on a regular basis, cover it with a bandage dressing, ideally with compression, and apply petroleum jelly to keep the area moist.

- If you need surgery, talk to your doctor about non-invasive or minimally invasive procedures.

What Happens If You Pop Your Own Keloid?

A keloid is not a pimple that can be popped on your own! In fact, physicians advise against doing so since you risk contracting an infection and worsen the issue. You can either try one of the home remedies mentioned above or visit your dermatologist for the best treatment option for your situation.

Conclusion

Keloids are the result of an extreme version of the body's natural scar tissue processes.

Keloids can be considerably reduced in size and pigmentation with natural therapies, making them less apparent. Home remedies are very helpful right after a wound, puncture, or burn. If home remedies do not improve the keloids, visit a doctor about all available choices. They might advise you to use over-the-counter or prescription lotions and gels. If other treatments fail, surgery and laser removal are viable options. Remember that

keloids can reappear no matter
what treatment is utilized to treat
them.